Whinchat's First Adventure

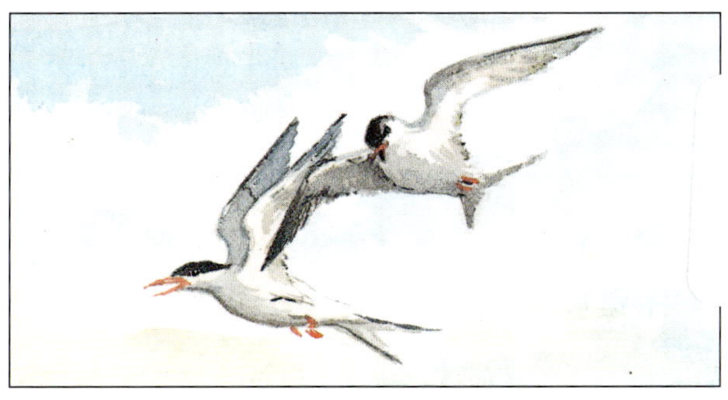

Written by Carole Frances Hughes

Illustrated by Alan Padwick O.B.E.

OPUS BOOK PUBLISHING LIMITED

Acknowledgements
Medina Valley Centre, Newport, Isle of Wight
John Claridge Boatbuilders of Lymington

First Published 1998 by Opus Book Publishing Limited

Printed in Hong Kong through World Print Ltd
Book design by Indigo

Opus Book Publishing Limited

It's nearly Spring

Alan Brown reached for another slice of his wife's sticky fruit cake. "Delicious" he commented, with his mouth half full! The twins, who were eight, were eating large hunks of farmhouse bread, covered with peanut butter. Soda, their 2 year old springer spaniel, hovered near their father's feet - she also loved fruit cake!

It was a beautiful day in late March. The garden was full of daffodils and crocus. Spring came early on the island. The family were eating tea in the sun-room and they could just see their Lymington Scow, Whistler, in the garden.

Alan Brown had been away working in Saudi Arabia for over a year. He stood up to look at Whistler as she sat, snug in her blue canvas cover on a launching trolley. "It's rained a lot this month, Whistler probably needs bailing out, " he observed.

Suzie, who was two hours older than her brother Rupert, looked at her father. "When are you going to teach us how to steer Whistler?" she asked.

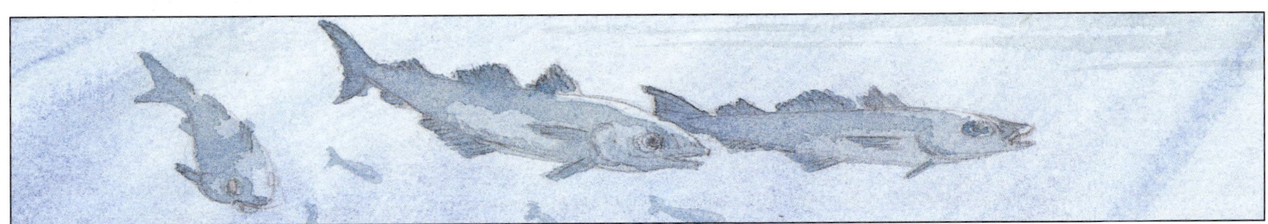

"More tea darling?" Sarah Brown asked her husband.

"Suzie, you and Rupert are old enough to attend an 'Oppie' course at the local Sailing Centre. I'll phone them later and see when their next course is."

"Wow!" exclaimed Suzie.

"What's an 'Oppie'?" Rupert asked.

"It's the perfect small dinghy to learn to helm in - can be made from wood or fibreglass, with just one sail. It's really called an Optimist" explained their father.

"Can two of us sail in an 'Oppie' ?"asked Suzie.

"You might just fit in, but if you do a course you would learn how to sail single-handed. There would be instructors with you, following you round in safety boats."

"When would they do the course?" asked the twins' mother.

"In the school holidays. I'll probably phone tomorrow and see if there's a course planned for half-term."

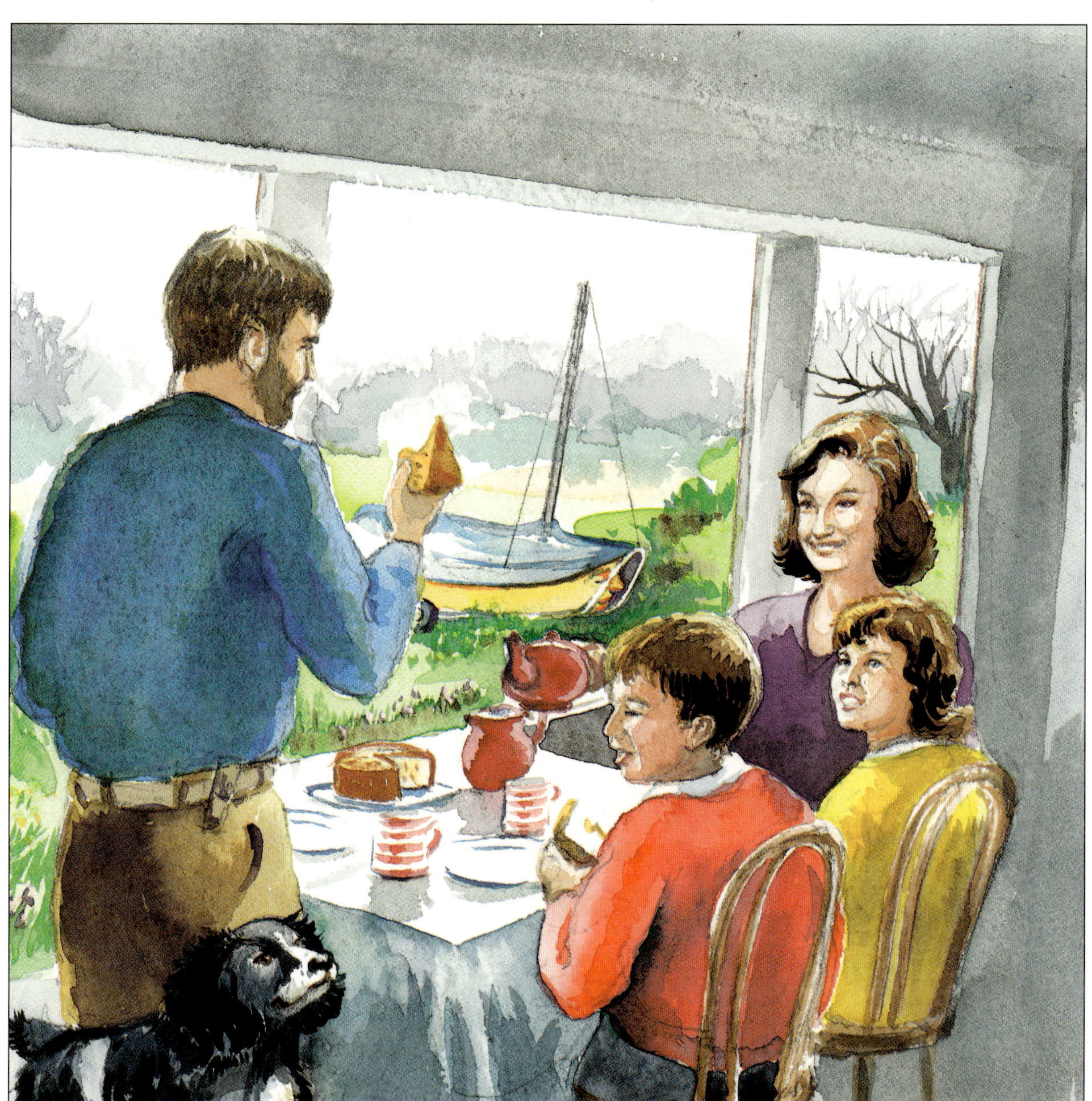

Alan Brown looked pleased. He had missed sailing in the sheltered waters of Shalfleet and Newtown. He knew how much fun the twins would have if they were properly taught. He gave Suzie a big smile.

Suzie, who wanted to tell Whistler about this plan, excused herself, opened the french windows and jumped onto the patio.

Whistler was half asleep. She always slept a lot when little was happening. Little had happened for a long time!

"Wake-up, Whistler, I've something important to tell you." Suzie tapped on the little dinghy's side. Whistler half-opened her eyes and looked at Suzie.

"It's too cold to go sailing," she observed in a sleepy and slow voice.

"Daddy is going to send us on an 'Oppie' course," announced Suzie, hopping up and down to keep warm. The easterly wind was chilly!

"I don't want to go on an 'Oppie' course," Whistler replied, closing her eyes again.

"Not you, silly, Rupert and me!"

"Fine, fine" muttered the little yellow boat, as she settled down for another snooze - then she sneezed!

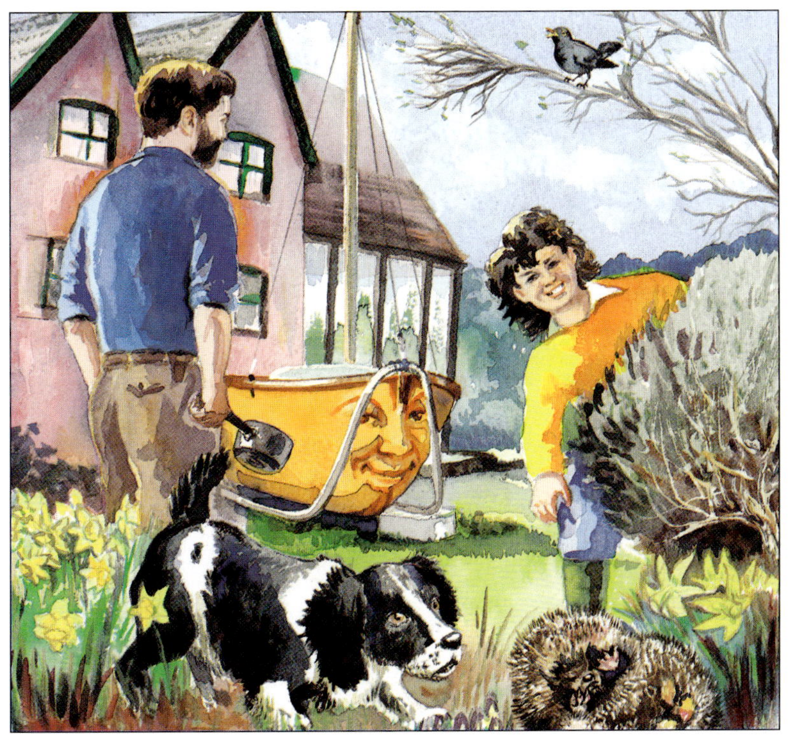

"You've probably caught cold!" said Suzie. She lifted a corner of the blue cover and peered inside. "Your floorboards are floating again!"

Suzie let herself back into the sun-room. "Whistler's full of water and she's very cold," she told her father.

Half an hour later, Whistler was a lot drier. Her cover was off and all the rain water had gone. Alan Brown put down the saucepan he had used as a bailer.

"Poor Whistler" he observed, "I've a lot of work to do on your woodwork - your mast needs rubbing right back and re-varnishing."

Whistler looked pleased. Her eyes opened and she smiled, but she said nothing. Talking boats only talk to children!

Suzie skipped onto the lawn. She had spotted Dozey, their resident hedgehog, under a lavender bush. So had Soda!

"Woof, woof, woof," she barked, springing from one side of the bush to the other - her long ears flying as she jumped.

"Woof, woof." Dozey moved slightly but refused to unroll from a tight prickly ball. Soda poked her nose a little nearer and put out a paw. Then she sprang back in surprise and sat down and licked her paw.

Suzie laughed. "Poor Soda" she commented, "you should know hedgehogs are prickly." She poked Dozey gently with a small stick.

"Wake up, Dozey," she said, "it's nearly Spring."

A blackbird trilled in agreement and all the daffodils nodded their heads.

Whistler went back to sleep.

The 'Oppie' Course

'What are you doing, Rupert?" Suzie was only half-awake, but she could hear her twin brother unzipping his rucksack.

"I'm just checking my sailing things." Rupert had the tidy mind and knew about checking lists!

> cotton jumper
> spare jeans
> pair of spare socks (and pants)
> pair of sailing shoes or plimsolls
> towel (just in case)
> waterproof top (lightweight)
> sun hat (peaked)
> sun cream and lip salve

"You know it's all there," said Suzie, sitting up in bed, "Mum packed for you."

"I just want to be certain" said Rupert, climbing back into his bunk bed.

"Night Suzie."

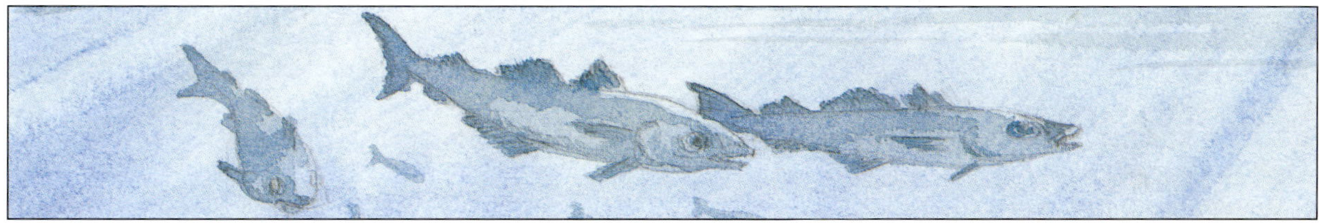

At 9.30 am the next morning they were standing outside the Sailing Centre - watching other children arriving and looking past the modern buildings towards the bank of the river Medina.

"Look," said Suzie, "there are some dinghies by the pontoon, perhaps they're 'Oppies'."

"No," said a friendly voice behind her. "They're a lot bigger and are called Seastars." It was Alex, the Centre's host. Half an hour later, Suzie and Rupert, together with eight other children, were fitted out with buoyancy aids. These were adjusted for tightness.

Their introductory sail was on a Seastar, a 16' fibreglass dinghy built by the Centre's boatyard for teaching sailing. Their instructor, Charles, explained how you get into and move about in a boat. He also told them that they would wear helmets in the Optimists in strong (force 3+) winds. Then they were towed by a safety boat to a wider part of the river. For the next hour they tacked backwards and forwards with Charles telling them to 'duck' every time the boom went across.

He explained what the Seastar's centreboard was for. "It makes the boat go straight," he said "but when you get into shallow water you have to pull it up."

They found that when the mainsail was pulled in using the mainsheet, the boat leaned over and when the sail was let out the boat came more upright again.

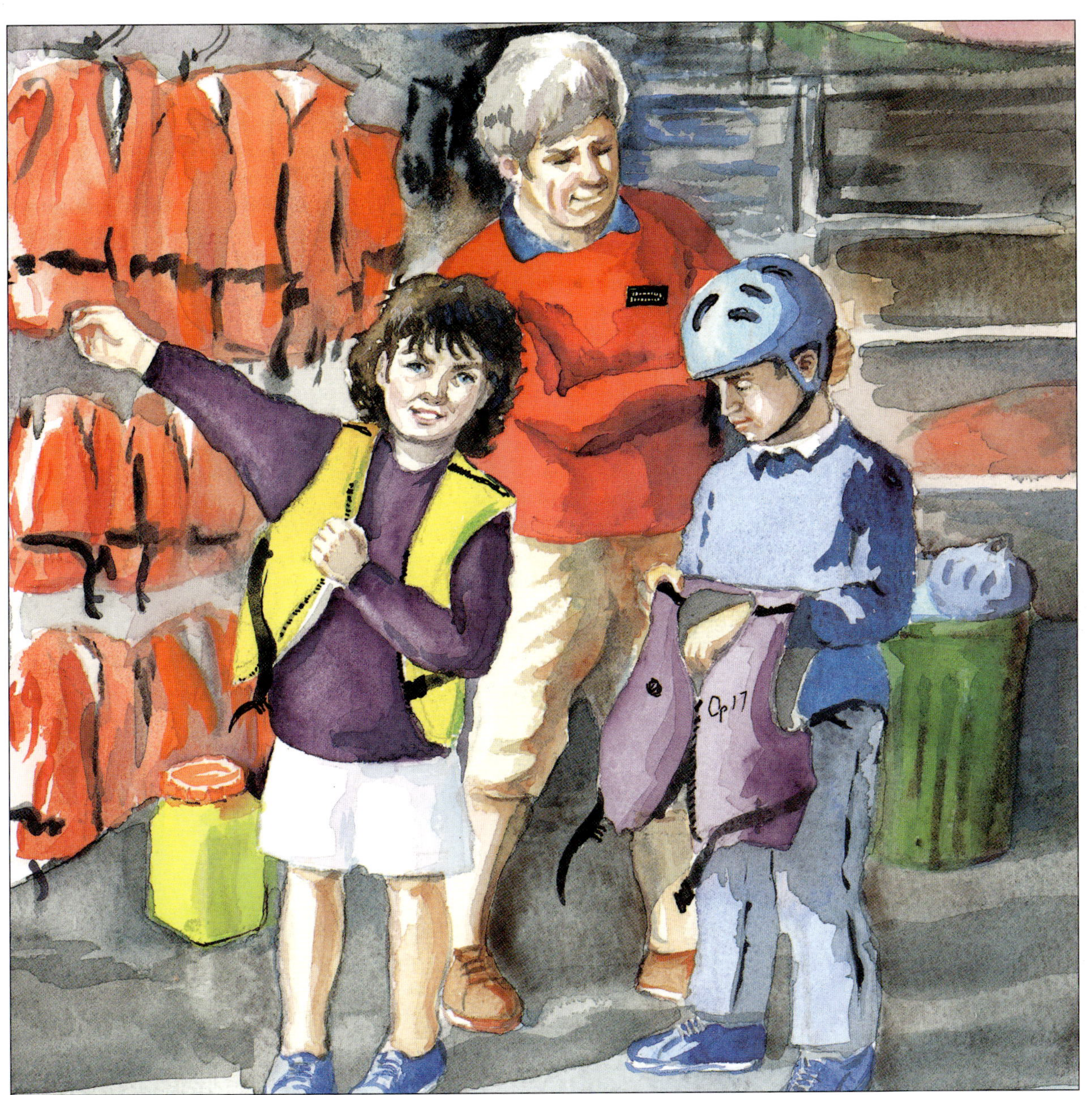

When the wind was behind the boat the sail was let right out. "This is called 'running'," explained Charles. They were allowed to help hold the tiller. It was quite exciting.

That afternoon the tide was out, so they all did practical work in one of the classrooms. They learnt a very useful knot called a bowline. Suzie found this quite difficult. They played with tiny models of yachts and learnt how to turn the little boats by putting the bow through the wind. That's called 'tacking'. Then they made their boats 'heave to' by tacking, but not letting the jib go.

They were shown their RYA Young Sailors Log Book and told that everything on the list would need to be ticked off, if they wanted to earn their Stage I and II Sailing Certificates.

The next day was their first introduction to an Optimist. It was quite windy, so they all put on safety helmets and adjusted them at the back for tightness. Then they put on their buoyancy aids.

First they learnt how to stand up and move around the 8' dinghy while it was tied up to the pontoon. This helps to build up confidence. Suzie felt happy but Rupert was a little less confident. There were lots of patient instructors watching every move the children made.

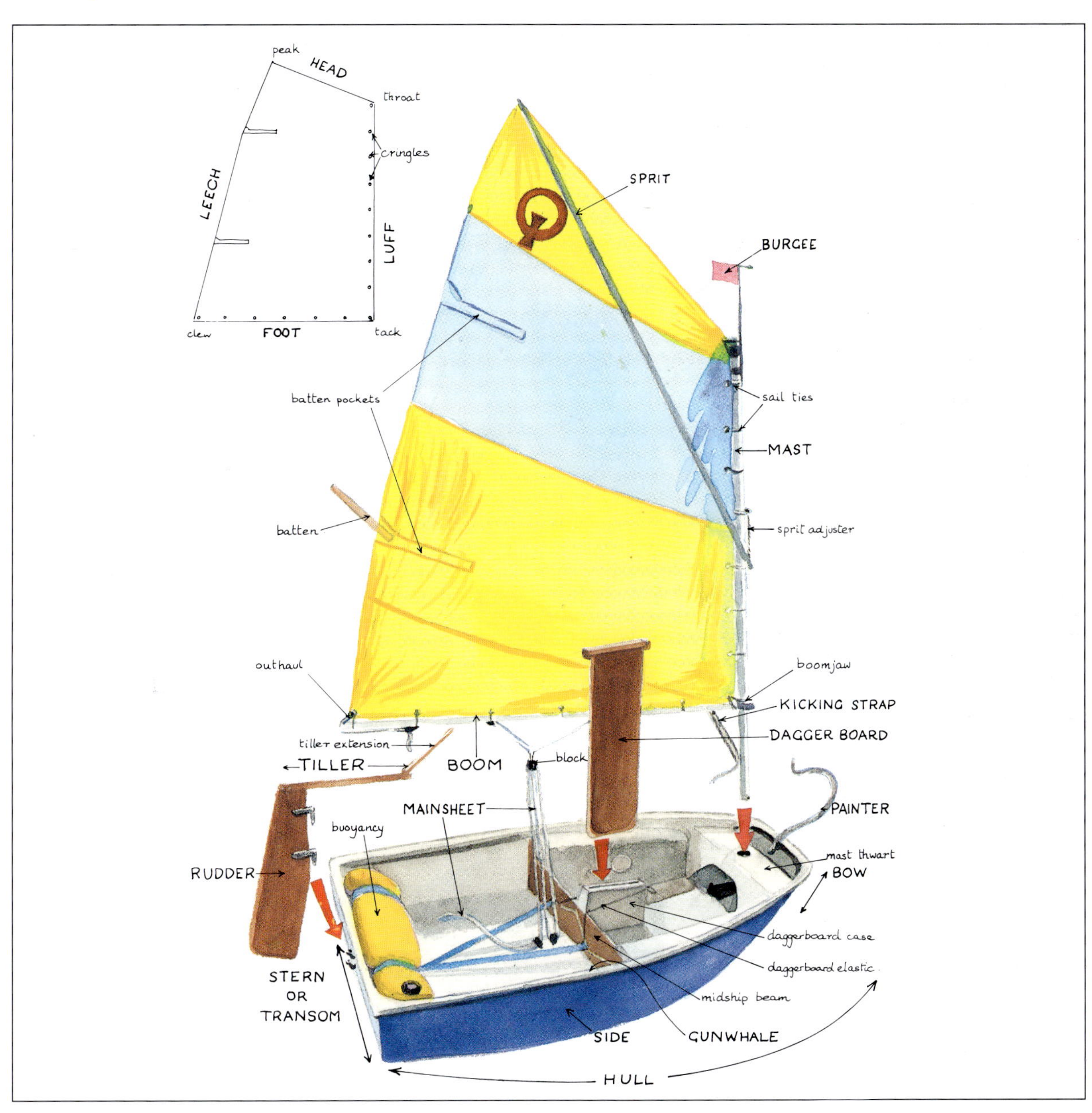

peak
HEAD
throat
cringles
LEECH
LUFF
clew
FOOT
tack
SPRIT
BURGEE
sail ties
MAST
batten pockets
sprit adjuster
batten
outhaul
boomjaw
KICKING STRAP
DAGGER BOARD
tiller extension
boom
block
PAINTER
TILLER
BOOM
MAINSHEET
buoyancy
mast thwart
BOW
RUDDER
daggerboard case
daggerboard elastic
STERN
OR
TRANSOM
midship beam
SIDE
GUNWHALE
HULL

Rupert helped unfurl the yellow and blue sail. "It isn't very big" he commented.

"That's because the sprit still has to go in to make it higher," explained Steve, the chief instructor. "When it's very windy we don't use it, so the sail is smaller."

One of the launches was anchored about 50 metres away. "Go on Suzie, sail to the launch. Pull in the mainsheet and you'll begin to move."

Suzie looked at the white launch, pulled in the mainsheet and felt the little boat gather speed. When she reached the launch, Charles called "push the tiller away from you and duck, then change sides - well done Suzie!"

Then it was Rupert's turn. "Don't wiggle the stick so much Rupert and look where you're going." Rupert's course was a bit of an S shape!

The days passed very quickly. They learnt what is meant by a 'gybe' and how to 'get out of irons'. This is when you aren't moving! Each time they successfully completed a part of their certificate, their instructor signed their log book.

Every evening Rupert and Suzie returned home with a different set of salty tales and occasionally a new bruise! They also developed big appetites!

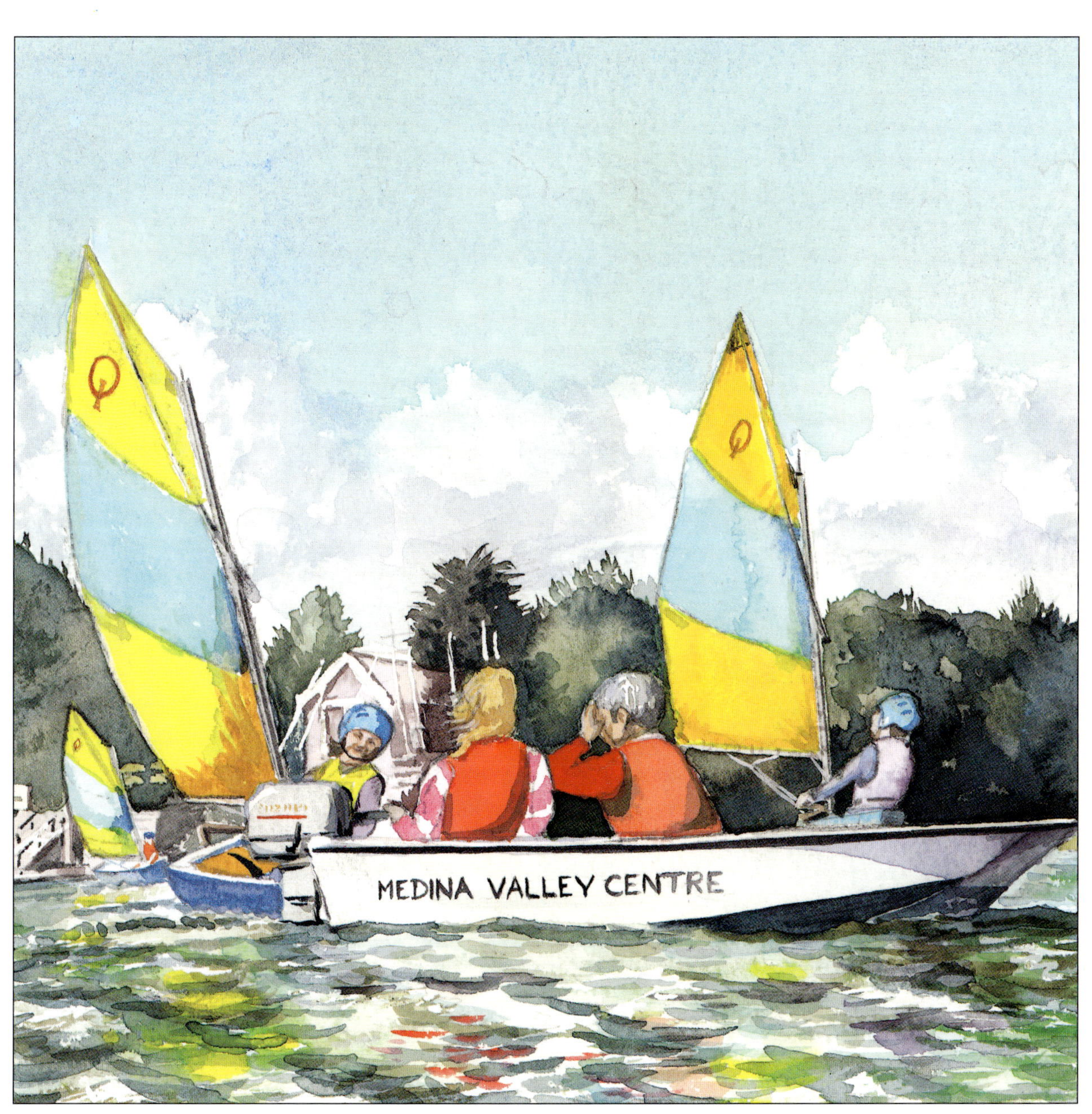

MEDINA VALLEY CENTRE

Gybing

(Turning the stern through the wind.)

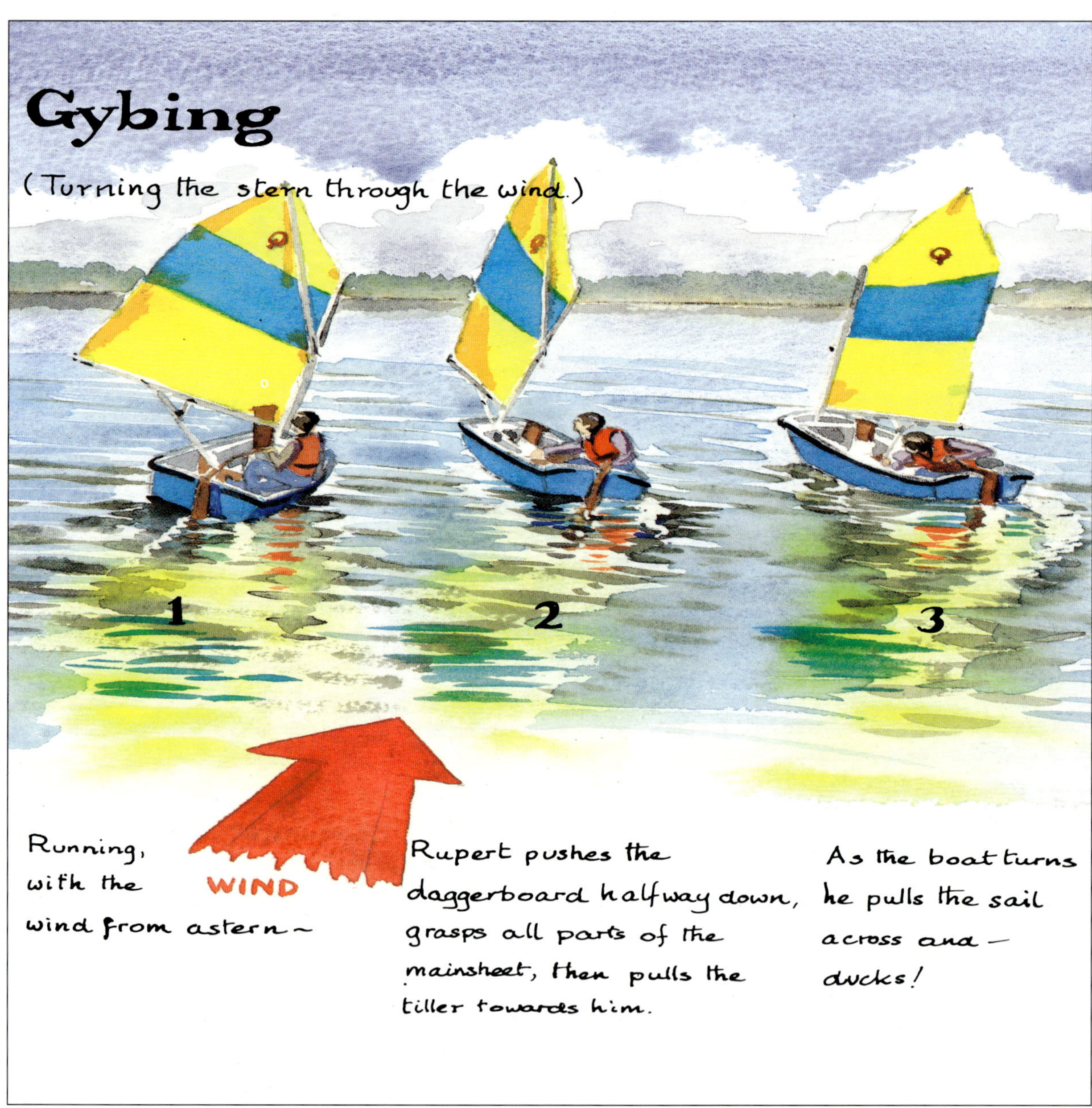

Running, with the wind from astern —

Rupert pushes the daggerboard halfway down, grasps all parts of the mainsheet, then pulls the tiller towards him.

As the boat turns he pulls the sail across and — ducks!

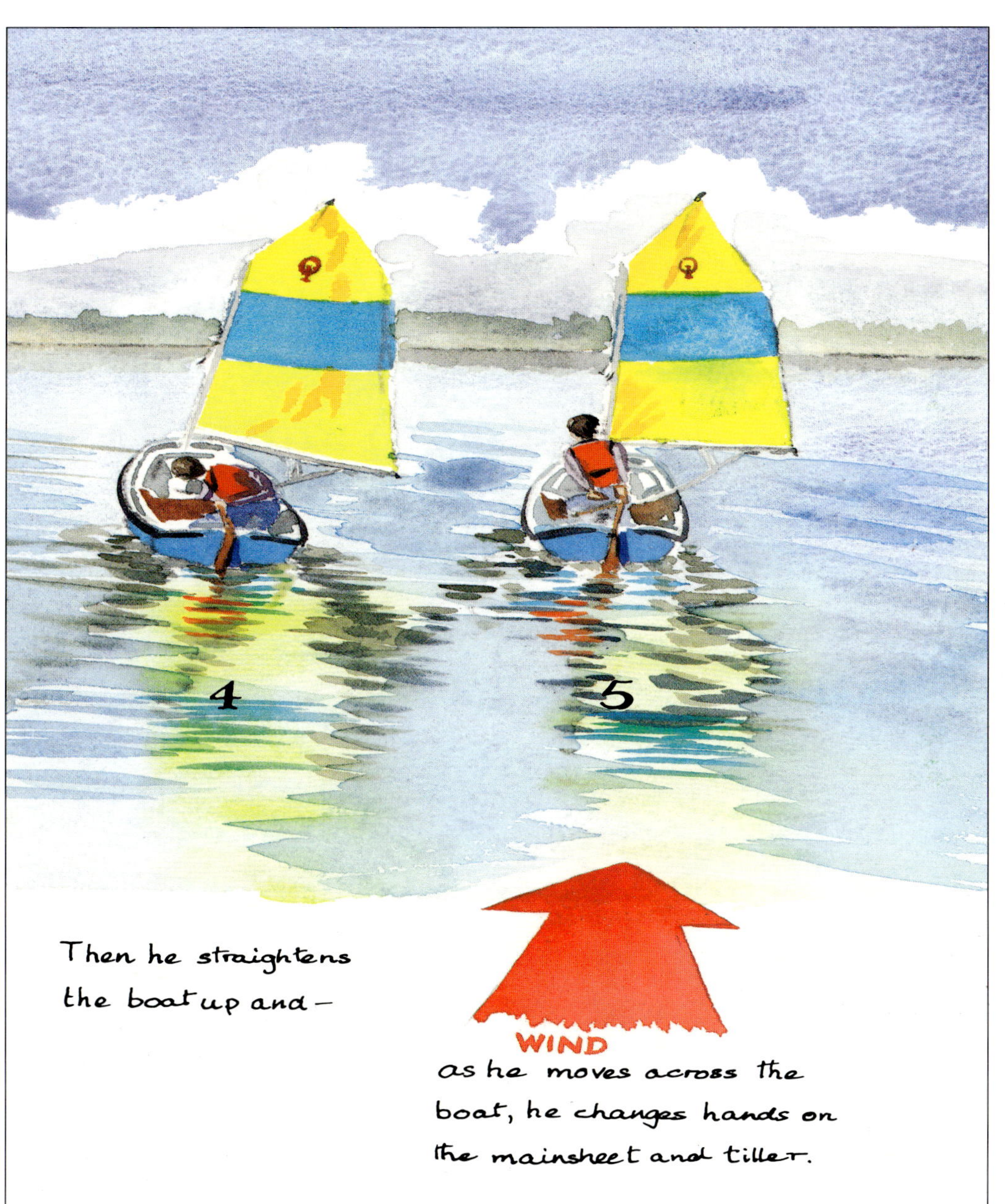

Then he straightens
the boat up and —

As he moves across the
boat, he changes hands on
the mainsheet and tiller.

On the Thursday they were due to capsize the 'Oppies'. As it was only the summer half-term holiday, the water was still very cold. Alan Brown saw the expression on his wife's face.

"They have to start learning this - it does happen," he explained. "I'm sure they won't be in the water long and I know they take a hot shower afterwards."

Capsizing is when the boat heels too far and tips over. This can happen in strong winds. Lesson 1 is **ALWAYS STAY WITH THE BOAT**.

It was a very quick practice and done with the Optimist firmly tied up to the pontoon. A dry Rupert suddenly found himself in some very cold water!

"Hold onto the mainsheet and swim round the stern of the boat" he was instructed. "Now hold onto the daggerboard and lean on it." As the Optimist came upright Rupert was told to clamber in and bail (scoop) out the water. Once the water has gone the 'Oppie' can be sailed again. Rupert took his dripping body off for a shower. Thank goodness that's over, he thought, I had collywobbles thinking about it!

The best moment of the week was when they were presented with their RYA Start Sailing Stage II Certificate. Two very proud and wind-tanned children returned home to a celebration tea, with chocolate fudge cake.

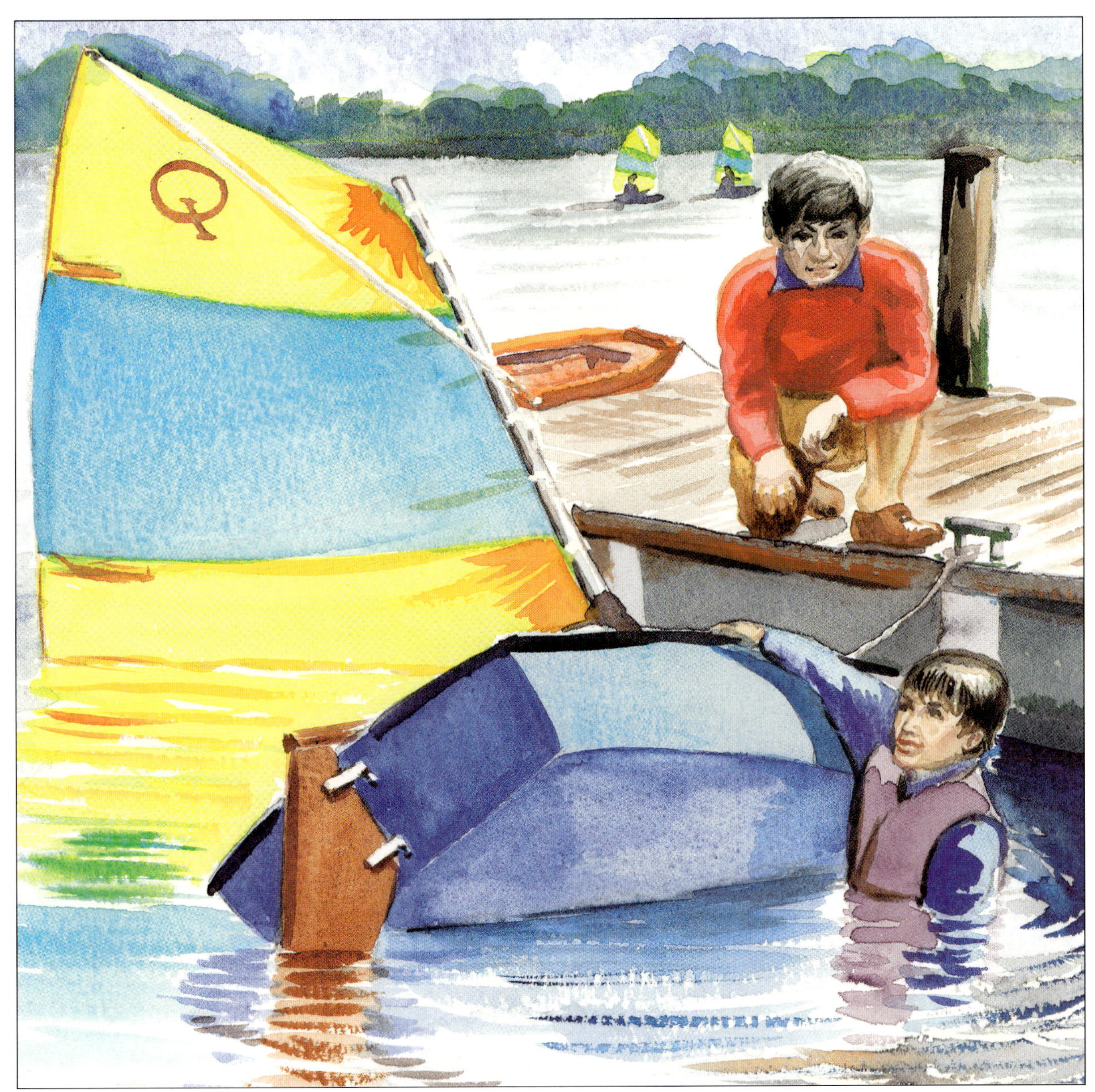

"Look Whistler," a tousled Suzie waved her important certificate. "I've passed my Stage II and so has Rupert."

Whistler actually looked quite pleased, for she had been scrubbed and polished and a new coat of varnish now made her wooden gunwhale and mast gleam.

"What's a Stage II?" she asked Suzie.

"It's proof that we've done things like tacking, gybing and even a practise capsize."

"What's a capsize?" asked Whistler.

"It's when you're tipped into the water and it was very cold water" explained Suzie, trying to remember everything she had been told. "You have to stay with the boat and get it upright by leaning on the daggerboard."

"I've never quite capsized and if I did I've got built-in buoyancy tanks." - Whistler was getting technical!

"Tea's ready, Suzie" her father called from the sun-room.

I wonder what plans and surprises he has in store for Rupert, Suzie and Whistler!

Hullo Whinchat

Rupert woke early. A duck was quacking on the lawn that ran down to the creek. Soda woke and barked to get out, she loved chasing ducks!

Rupert opened his bedroom window and leaned out. It was the first day of the summer holidays and his father had promised a surprise. They had sailed on Whistler twice since the 'Oppie' course. Both Rupert and Suzie had wanted to steer and it was a squash when Soda came.

There wasn't a lot of water in the creek. Rupert could see Whistler by their little pontoon. Then he blinked, for there was a small white boat tied up next to their yellow scow.

"Suzie, wake-up, there's another boat by our pontoon."

Rupert was very excited. Suzie jumped down from her bunk and joined Rupert at the window. The door from the sun-room opened and their father emerged with Soda.

"Dad, Dad, we can see another boat," called Suzie.

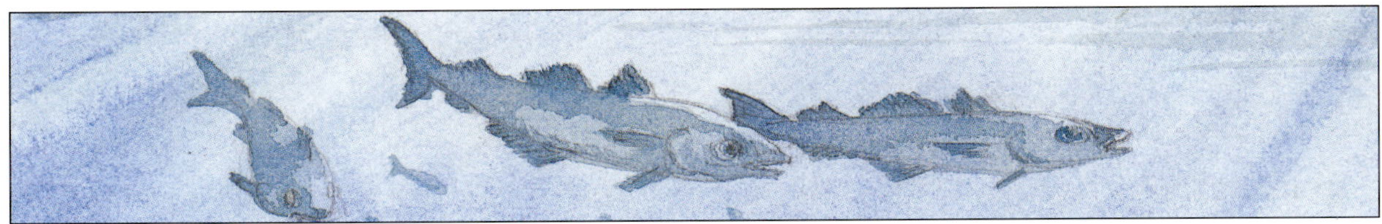

"Stop leaning out of the window, you two, get dressed and come and look," instructed their father.

The children threw on shorts and T shirts and raced downstairs. They ran, barefoot, down the damp grassy slope to the creek. Whistler had a new friend!

It was small and white and looked very familiar. It was a fibreglass 'Oppie', with a yellow buoyancy bag. Whistler was looking very smiley.

"Whistler, who's this?" asked Suzie.

"I'm Whinchat" replied the little boat, in a little voice!

At that moment Soda decided to create a rumpus! "Woof woof, woof woof woof."

"Quack quack, quack quack."

Soda, tail wagging furiously, was running, helter skelter after the ducks. The ducks flew into the air, with a final "Quack". Soda sat down - she looked very pleased with herself and her tongue lolled out of the corner of her smiley mouth.

"Breakfast everyone," called their mother, from the sun-room door. Over breakfast they talked about rigging Whinchat and carefully worked out the tides.

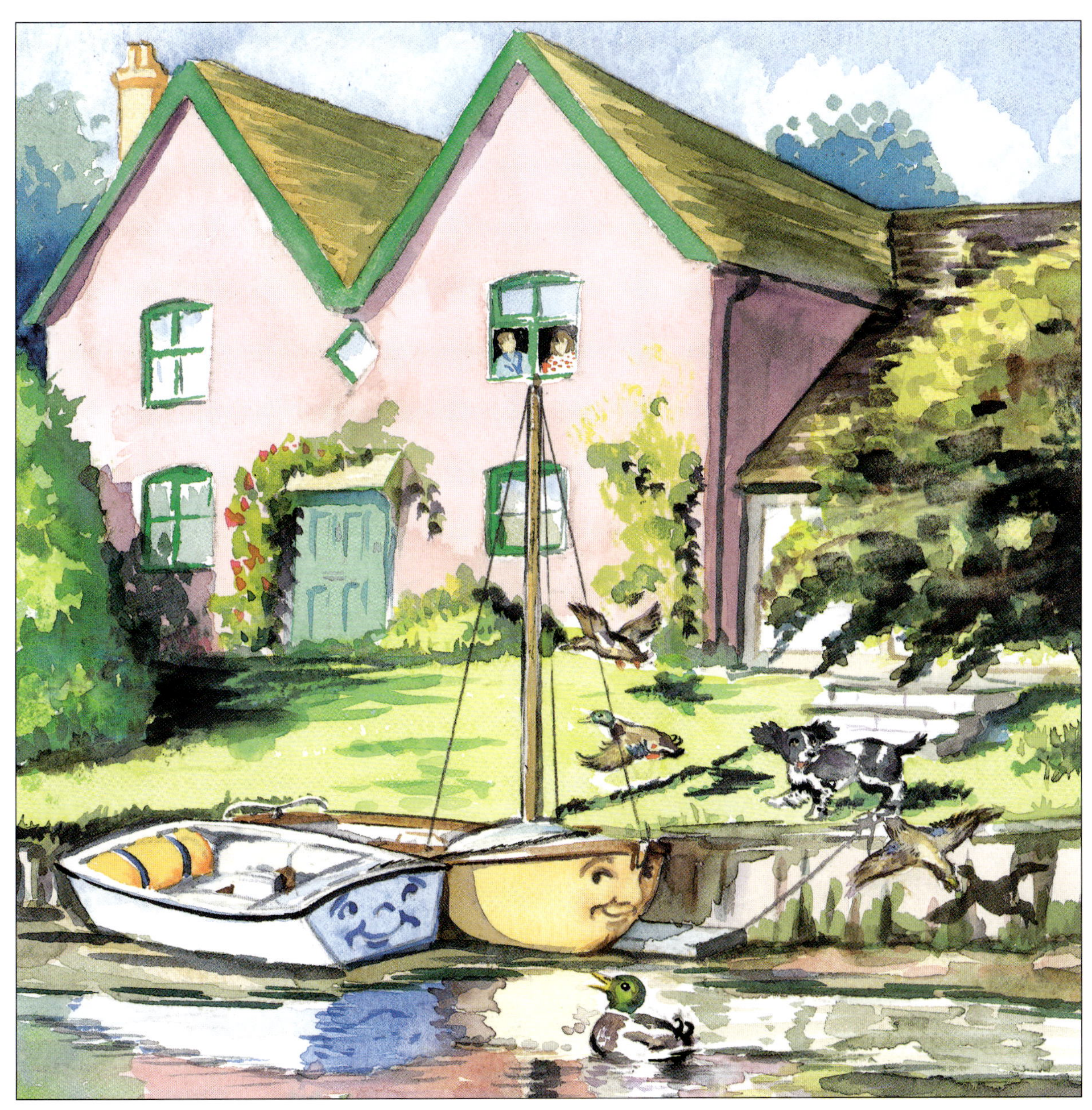

"We'll have to find somewhere else to keep the boats during the holidays" said Alan Brown. "It's hopeless here, we only get a couple of hours sailing before the tide's going the wrong way."

"What time can we go this morning?" asked Rupert, with his mouth half-full of toast and honey.

"Empty your mouth before you speak, dear," instructed his mother.

"High tide is at 1300 hours, (that's 1 o'clock) - this means we can leave just before it goes slack at noon and we ought to be on our way back just after 1400 hours, (that's 2 o'clock). Otherwise it will be running out too strongly," explained Rupert's father, looking at his tide chart. "If we meet at 1100 hours, (that's 11 o'clock), we can rig the two boats and be underway at slack tide."

"Shall I make some sandwiches?" asked Sarah Brown.

Her husband gave her a big smile. "Lots please love, and some drinks would be nice," he answered.

At 1100 hours the children were helping carry sails, battens, rudders, tillers and Whinchat's daggerboard and mast from the garage down to the creek. Whistler's centreboard stayed onboard. Then they collected paddles, bailers and buoyancy aids. There was a lot of gear! The children rigged Whinchat and their father rigged Whistler.

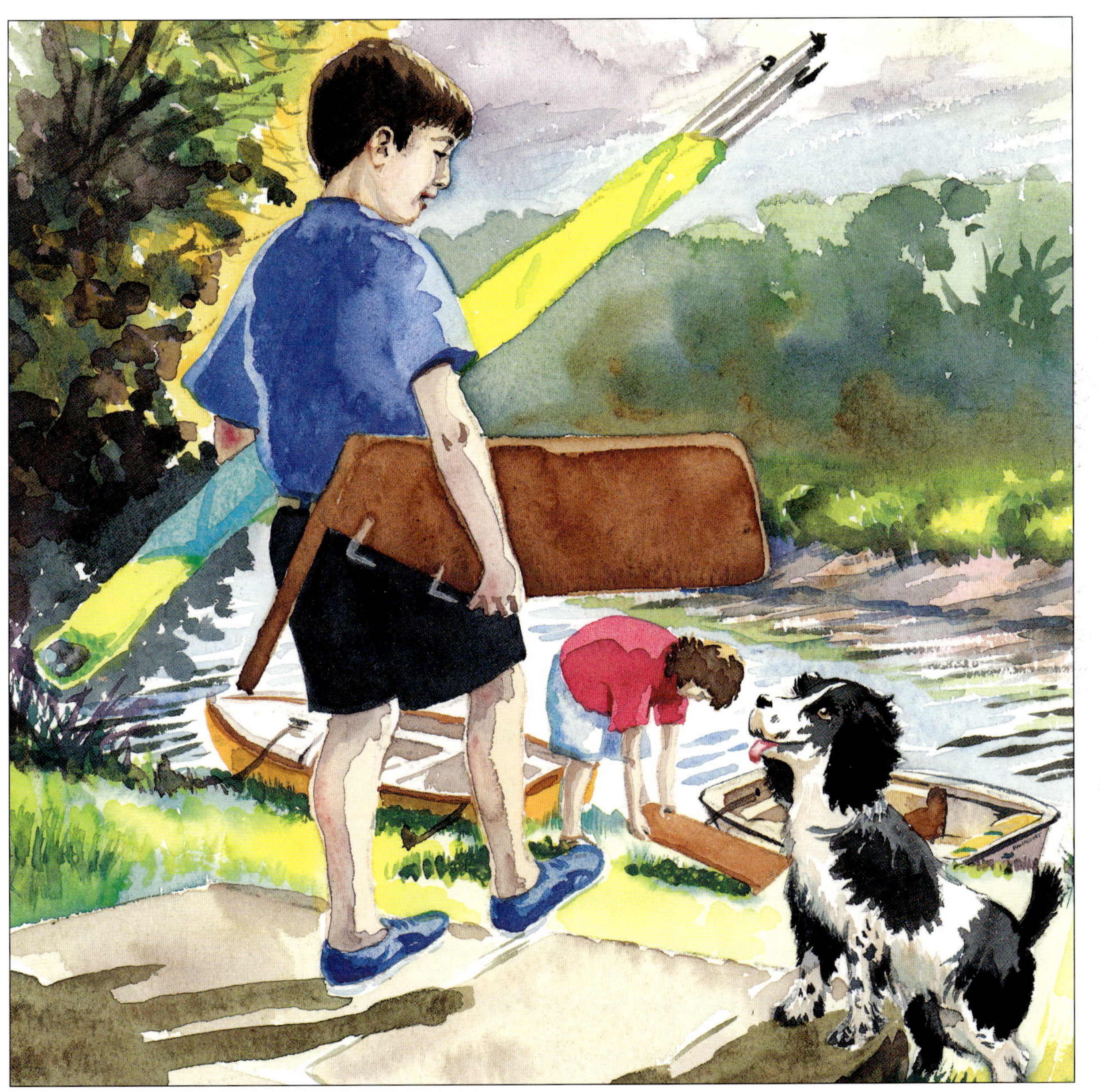

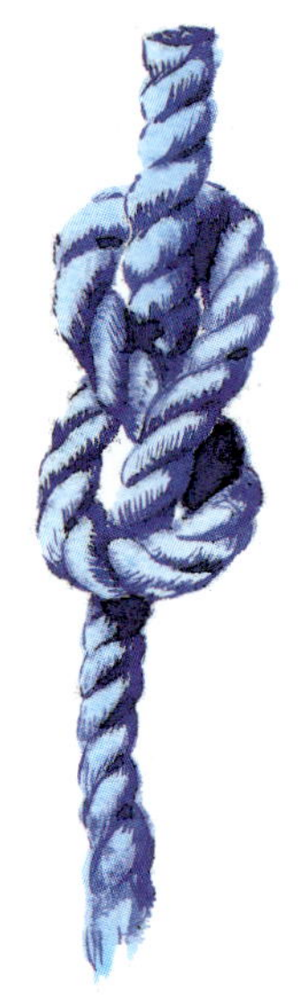

"What's this knot on the end of the mainsheet?" he asked Suzie, whilst undoing it!

"It's a figure of eight knot" replied Suzie.

"It looked like a thumb knot," her father laughed, "more knot practice needed, Suzie."

"What's a figure of eight knot used for?" asked Whinchat.

"Stopping ropes running through holes or blocks," explained Suzie.

"I haven't sailed before," explained Whinchat.

"That's alright, just follow me," said Whistler kindly.

"Bags I have first go on Whinchat" said Rupert.

"That's not fair" said Suzie.

"Suzie, you take Whinchat down the creek until you reach the Shalfleet Quay pontoon," said their father, "we'll meet there. Buoyancy aids on and check each others for tightness."

"There isn't a lot of wind" observed Suzie - Whinchat's sail was flapping gently.

"The wind is coming from behind at present, so ease (let out) sail as soon as you are settled."

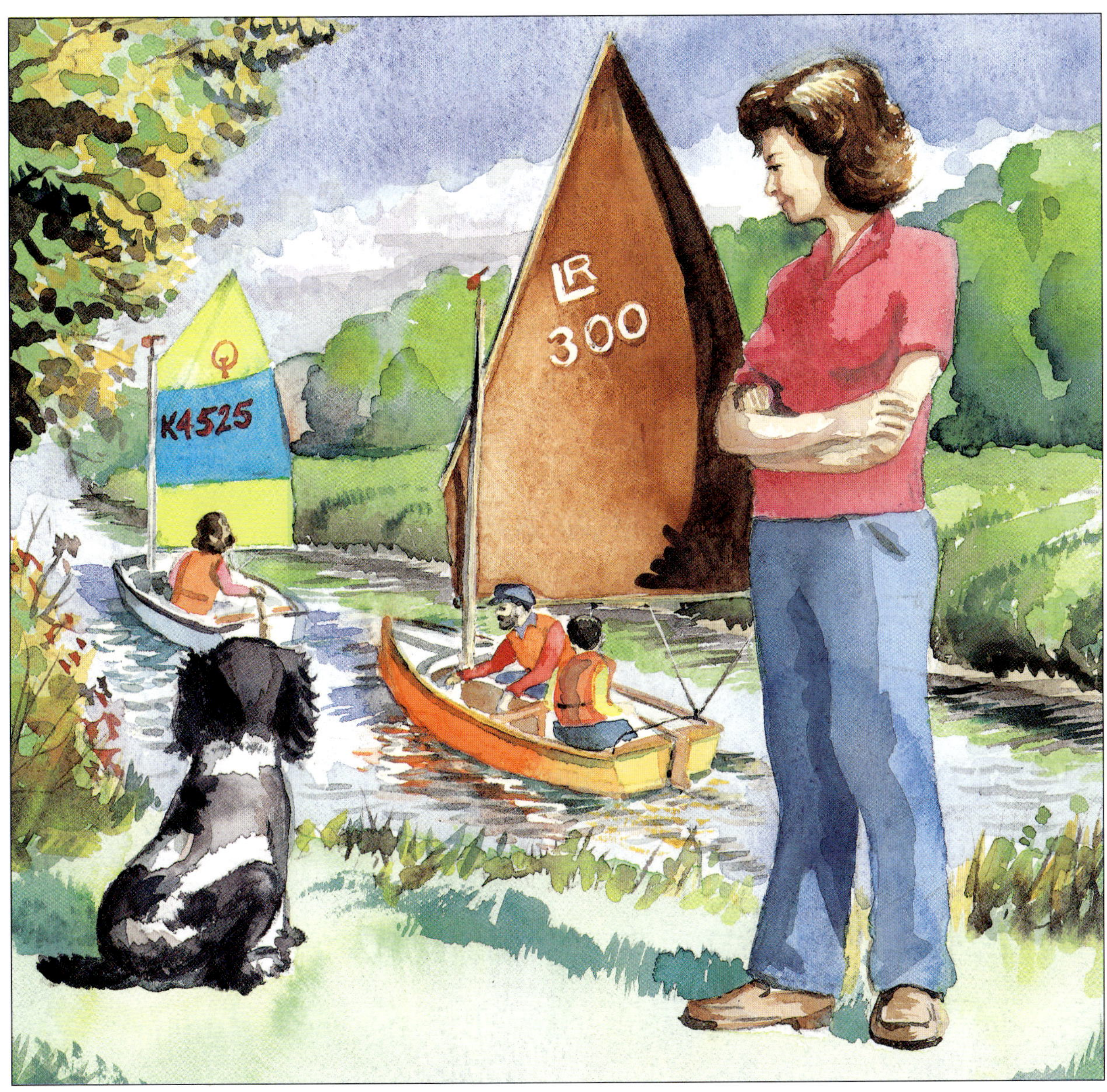
K4525
LR
300

Alan Brown gave firm orders. Suzie eased herself into the little boat, remembering to put her body weight in the right place. She sat down and let out the mainsheet. Rupert untied the little boat and gave it a slight push. Whinchat began to move and gave a little squeal "oooh!"

Rupert and his father got into Whistler and Rupert untied the painter. Soda barked and looked rather sad. She was to be left behind for Whinchat's first sail and her buoyancy aid had been left in the garage.

"Bye Soda," called Rupert, "we'll be back soon."

Soda whined a little, then scampered up the slope to join Sarah Brown, who had come into the garden to watch them leave.

The two dinghies sailed slowly along the narrow creek until the estuary widened. As it widened the wind increased a little. Suzie pulled in the mainsheet and the kicker as she steered the 'Oppie' closer to the wind.

Whinchat picked up speed. "Aaah!" said the little boat, hearing the water chuckling under her hull. A sudden gust of wind tipped the little 'Oppie' and Suzie had to move her bottom and lean back a little to stop Whinchat from heeling too far.

"Are you alright, Suzie?" called her father, looking back over his shoulder. Whistler, without her jib, was still faster than the Optimist.

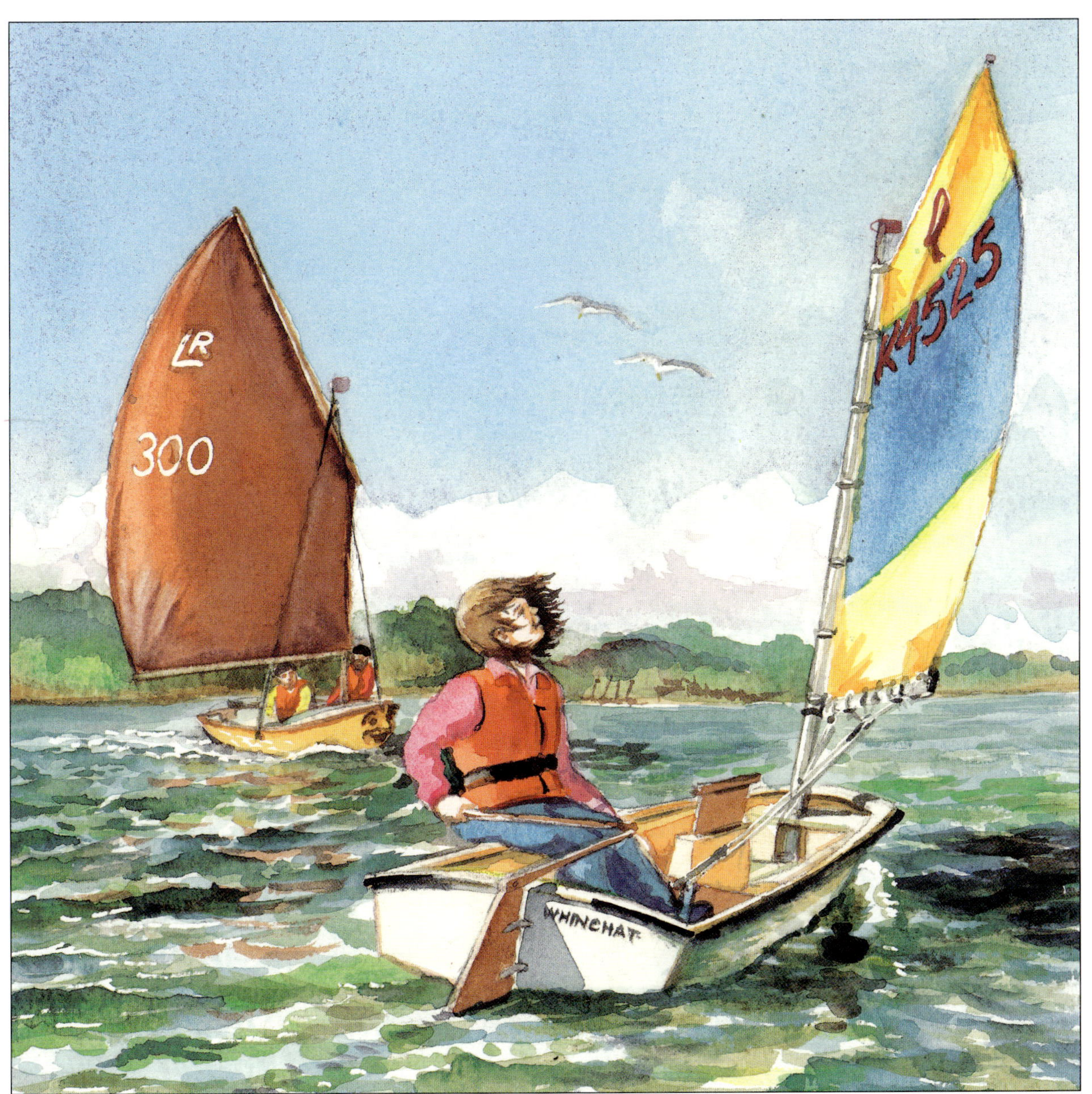

LR
300
R
K4525
WHINCHAT

"We're O.K.," replied Suzie, pointing Whinchat a little more downwind whilst easing the mainsheet.

"When you reach the pontoon, you'll need to let your sail right out and let it flap to spill the wind, before coming alongside," instructed her father.

"I know that," replied Suzie, but she was secretly pleased that she had been reminded of the correct way to approach the pontoon with a beam wind.

Whinchat approached the pontoon very slowly. Alan Brown was impressed. "Well done, Suzie" he said, as the little boat bumped gently against the pontoon. "We'll stow the sails while we have lunch."

"How do you like sailing, Whinchat?" asked Whistler.

"I like the chuckling noise the water makes when I move" said Whinchat.

"Chuckle, chuckle, chuckle," said Rupert, tying Whistler's painter to the pontoon.

"Can we have our sandwiches now, Dad? I'm hungry."

"So am I " agreed Suzie, "sailing always makes me ravenous. What kind of sandwiches are there?"

"Humans are always eating" commented Whistler, "they waste an awful lot of time on this eating habit!"

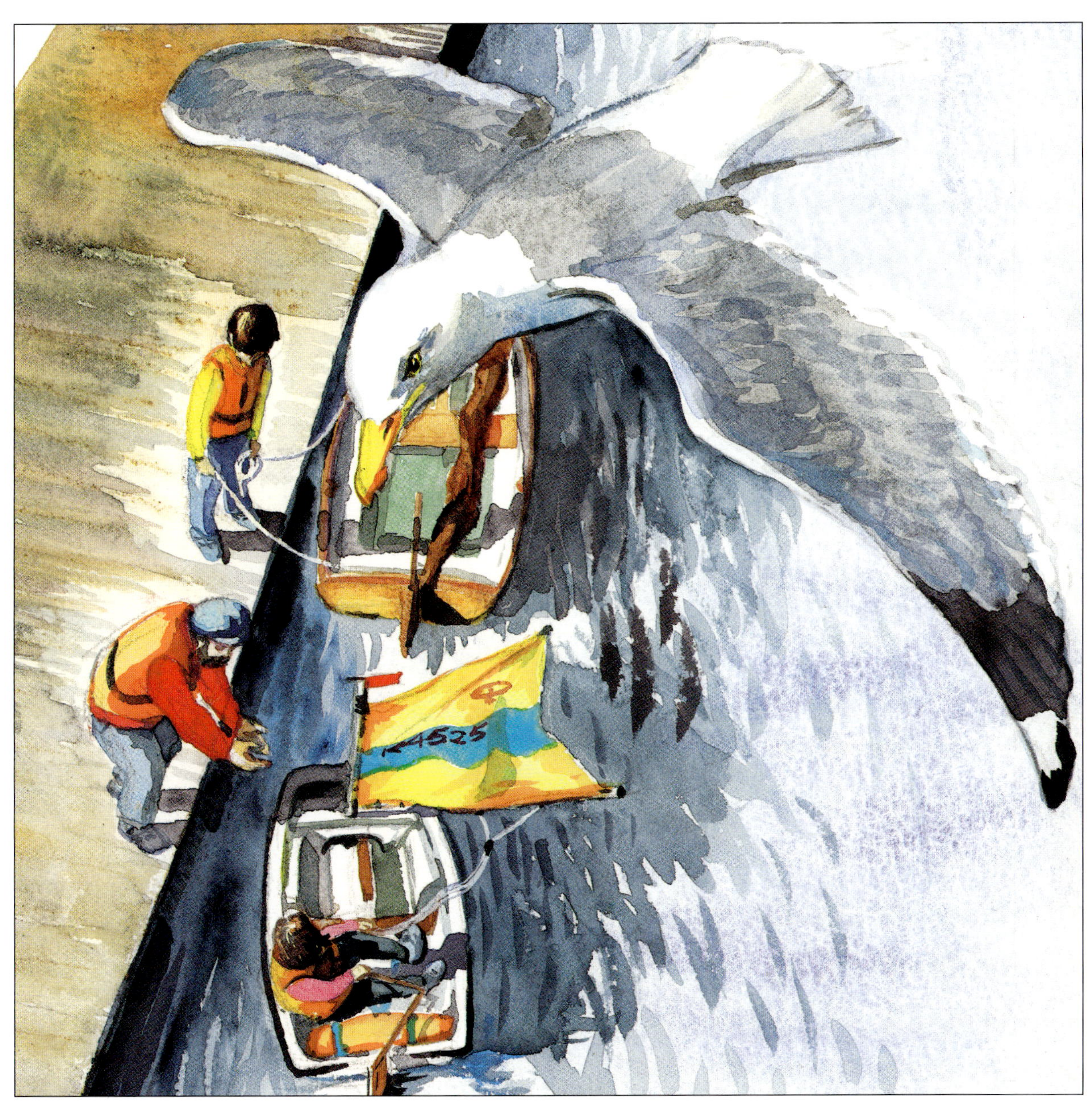
4525

Rupert laughed, "what kind of sandwich would you like, Whistler? Perhaps a fibreglass and bully beef sandwich?"

"What are you two burbling about?" asked their father, who, of course, couldn't hear the boats chatting.

"Get on with your sandwiches, we haven't a lot of time," instructed Whistler, who knew all about tides.

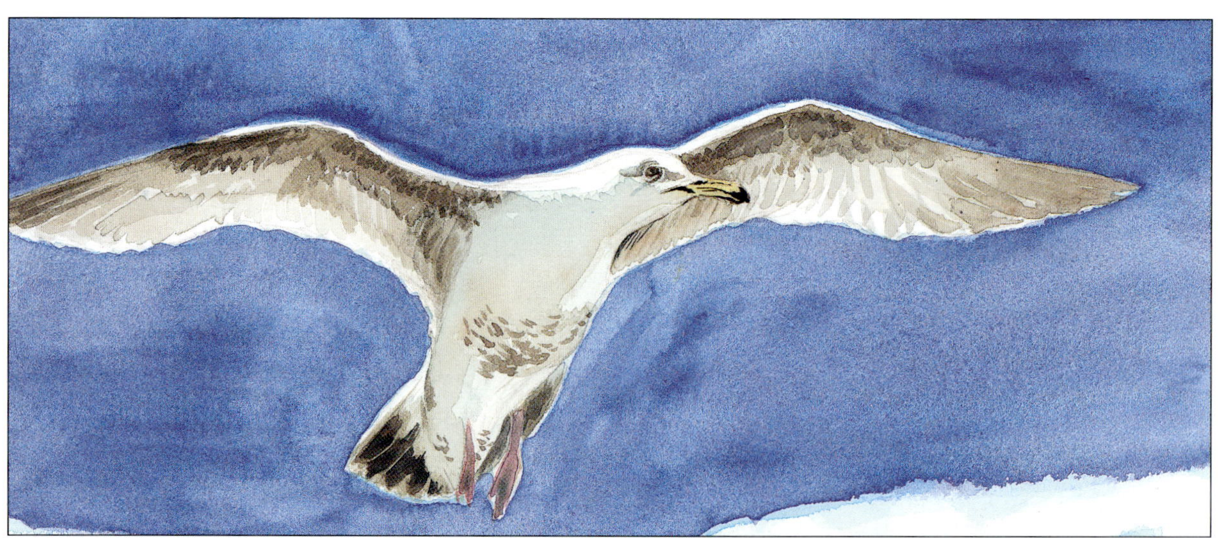

Whinchat's First Adventure

After the sandwiches and lemonade had been consumed, it was time for Rupert's go on Whinchat. She had been dozing in the warm sun, when suddenly Rupert was clambering aboard with little thought!

"Watch-out, Rupert," said Whistler, crossly, as the little boat tipped.

"Whoops" said Rupert, adjusting his weight to the centre of the 'Oppie' .

"Listen carefully, Rupert," ordered his father, "we've just over an hour of slack tide left, then it will begin to run out. This means we must soon be on our way home."

"Yes, Dad," said Rupert.

"It's now just after 1315 hours. I want you to be back here by 1345. What time is that?" asked Alan Brown.

"1.45." said Rupert, looking at his waterproof watch.

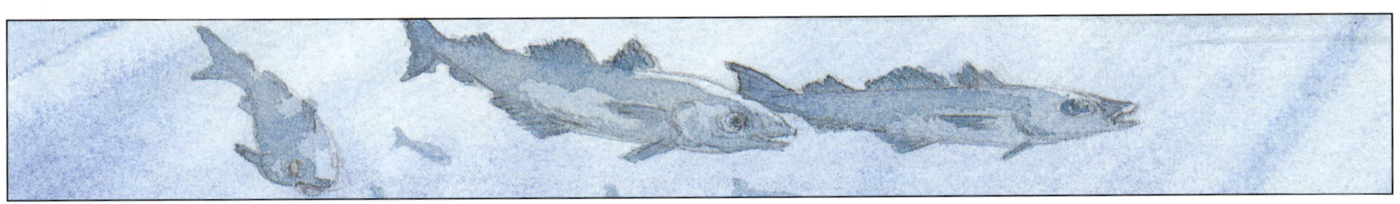

Suzie let go of the painter and her father gave Whinchat a push. Rupert pulled in the mainsheet and Whinchat sped away. The wind had veered (changed direction) a little and was blowing west sou'west.

Alan Brown untied Whistler's painter, ready to turn her round. The wind was now quite gusty.

"Oh no!"

He heard a sudden cry and turned to see Whinchat well heeled with Rupert not sitting out. Five seconds later Whinchat was experiencing her first capsize.

She was in a panic. "I'm going to sink!" she cried.

Rupert's head had appeared and he began to swim around the stern. "You won't sink, Whinchat," he told the little 'Oppie', "you have a buoyancy bag."

He pulled down the daggerboard, waited until the little boat turned into the wind, put his weight on the daggerboard, using his feet and heaved the little boat upright.

Whinchat was spluttering and going "oooh!" and finally "aah!" as she came upright, streaming with water.

Rupert pulled himself onboard, near the back of the boat and sat down. He let out the mainsheet and looked for the bailer. Then he realised that it had fallen out of Whinchat during the capsize. He saw it floating, with the paddle, about 10 metres away.

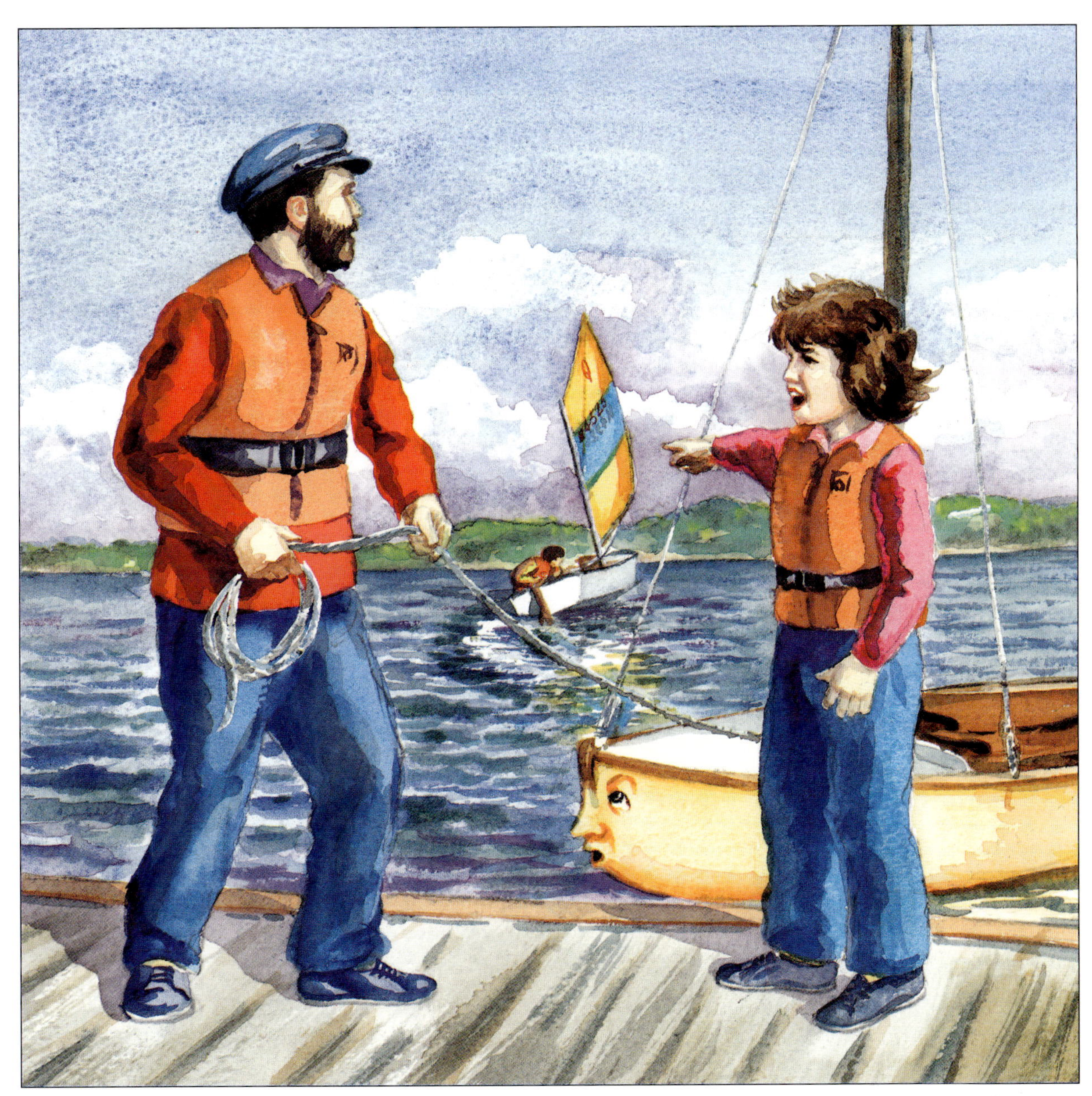

Meanwhile his father had dropped Whistler's sail again, got out the oars and was rowing toward the 'Oppie'.

"Dad, my bailer and paddle are floating away," shouted Rupert, prepared to go for another swim!

"Stay with the boat," instructed his father, "we're coming."

"Are you alright, Rupert?," asked his father, while Suzie leant across with Whistler's bailer. "Keep sitting while you bail and we'll retrieve your paddle."

"And bailer," said Whinchat, giving a small "hic!"

"When we get back we'll tow you to the pontoon and bail Whinchat out properly there," said Alan Brown.

Ten minutes later they were all safely back at the pontoon.

"What happened?" asked Suzie.

"It's my fault, I gybed rather suddenly and didn't shift my weight in time,"explained Rupert.

"The wind suddenly blew hard," added Whinchat still rather low in the water.

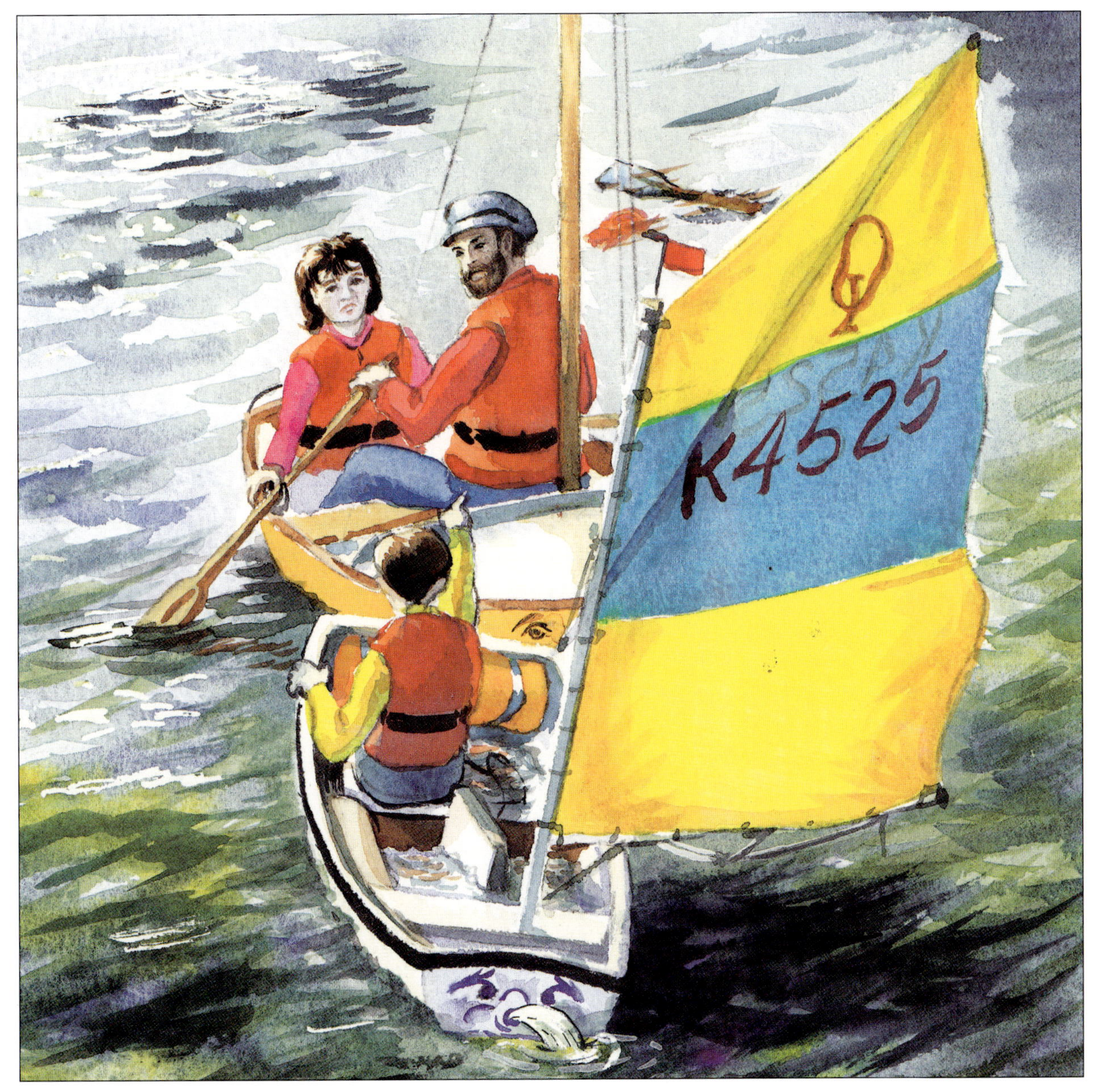
K4525

"Thank goodness for the capsize practice," commented Whistler, as Whinchat was bailed out.

When Whinchat had only a few inches of water left in her they set off. With the westerly wind on the beam it was a fast reach back to their home creek, but once they turned the corner into their narrow creek sailing was impossible. The wind was against them and the sails flapped uselessly. The tide was beginning to ebb and it was a hard row and paddle. At last, their little pontoon was in view.....

"Phew" said Rupert, "I'm steaming!" Rupert was sent off to have a hot bath, while Suzie and her father took down the sails and tidied the boats.

"We'll go and see the harbour master at Newtown tomorrow, Suzie, and see if they can find moorings there for Whistler and Whinchat," commented her father.

"Will that be better sailing?" asked Suzie.

"It will give us much more sailing time," explained her father, as they started to carry the gear up to the garage. After tea, Rupert decided to take a sponge to dry out Whinchat.

"How did you enjoy capsizing, Whinchat?" he asked the little boat, as he mopped out the water with the sponge.

"I didn't, I had hiccups all the way home," replied Whinchat.

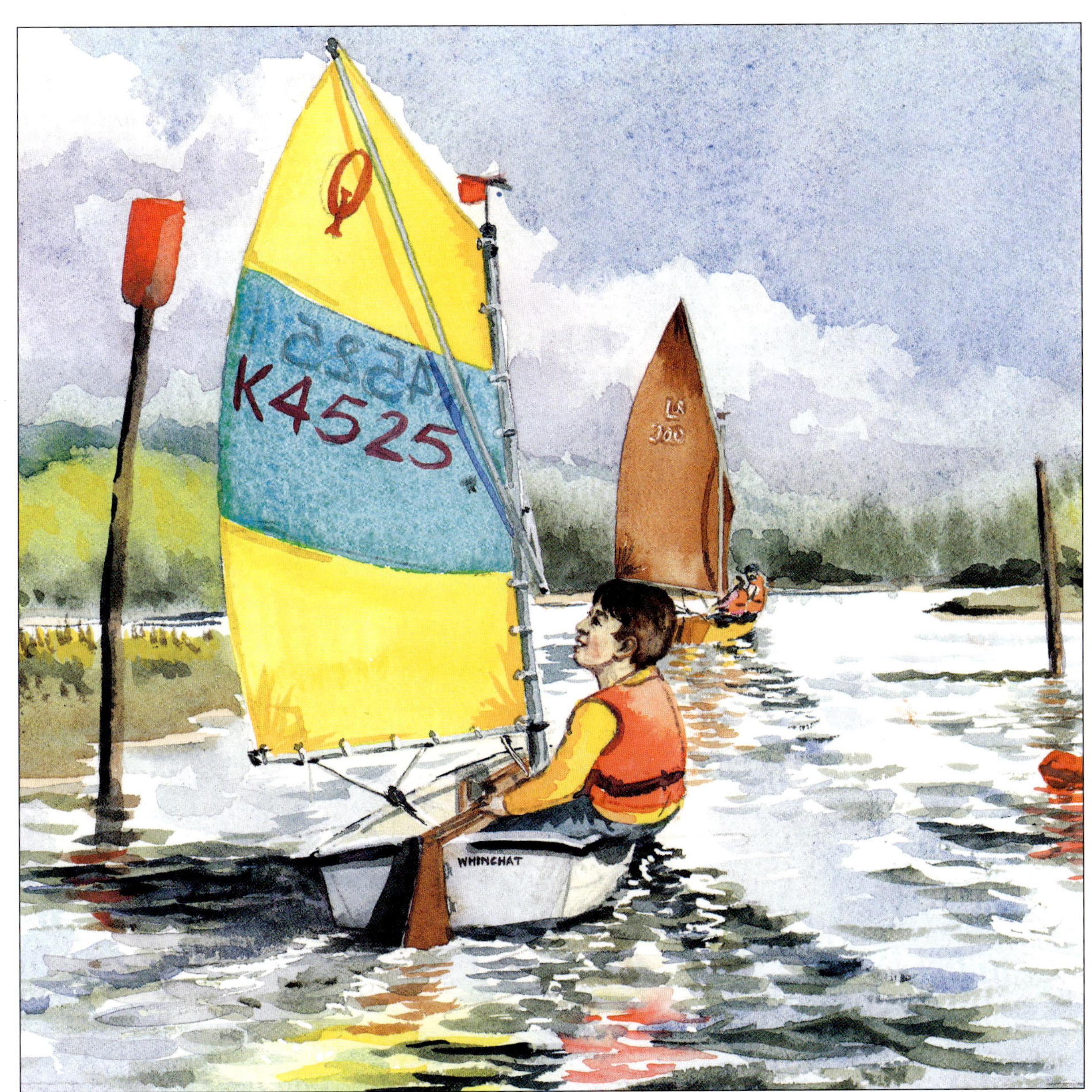

K4525
WHINCHAT

"Perhaps you'd better have a drink of water," suggested Whistler.

Have you ever heard boats giggle? Rupert left them both laughing and went to bed early.

It had been a tiring day.

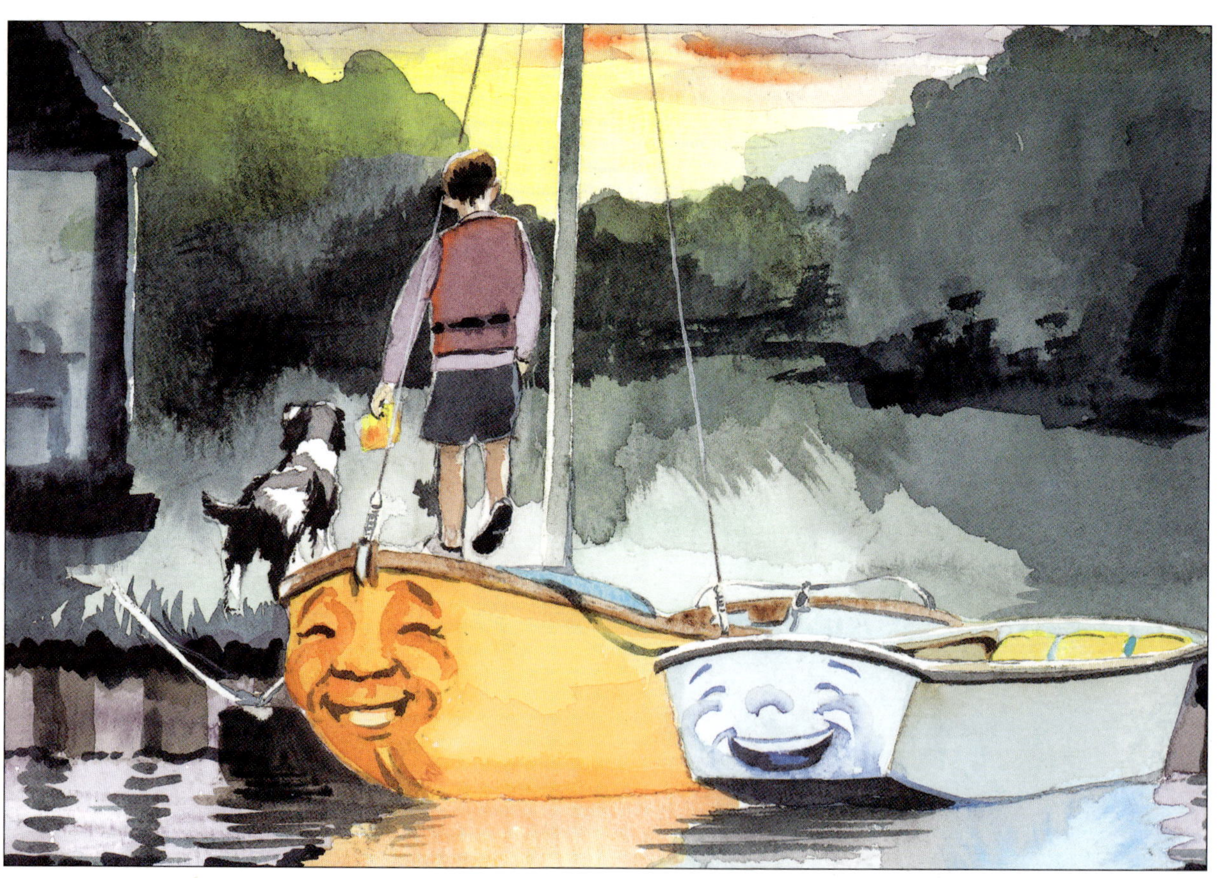